EPILEPSY AND CBD OIL

Epilepsy and CBD Oil:
What You Need to Know

DR. LOWELL BRAGG

Table of Contents

CHAPTER ONE

EPILEPSY AND CBD OIL

Epilepsy and CBD Oil: What You Need to Know

Cannabidiol (CBD) oil is a combination of CBD and a carrier oil. In the class of chemicals known as cannabinoids, CBD is one of many.

Although cannabidiol (CBD) oil has shown promise in the treatment of some epilepsy and seizure-related symptoms, the majority of patients still prefer to use the isolated CBD compound.

More permissive laws regarding cannabis in general have contributed to a recent uptick in study of cannabinoids like CBD.

It is important to discuss CBD oil with a doctor to determine if it is a good treatment option and to learn about any potential risks or side effects.

Read on to discover the many benefits of cannabis and CBD oil in the treatment of seizures.

Is it acceptable to use CBD in public?

Because of the passage of the Farm Bill in 2018, hemp is no longer considered to be the same thing as marijuana under the Controlled Substances Act. This made some hemp-derived CBD products with less than 0.3 percent THC federally legal. However, CBD products containing more than 0.3 percent THC still fall under the legal definition of marijuana, making them federally illegal but legal under some state laws. Be sure to check state laws, especially when traveling. However, the FDA has not yet approved CBD products for sale without a prescription, and the labels on some products may be misleading.

CHAPTER TWO

CBD oil: a brief explanation.

Research into the health benefits of CBD oil is ongoing.

CBD oil is a mixture of cannabidiol (CBD) and a carrier oil, such as olive, coconut, or other ingestible oils.

Cannabidiol is one of the main compounds in the cannabis plant. Tetrahydrocannabinol (THC), the compound most responsible for the psychoactive effects of cannabis, is the other major component.

Cannabidiol (CBD) is not psychoactive and will not result in the altered states of consciousness commonly associated with cannabis use.

However, some CBD oils that manufacturers label as full-spectrum or broad-spectrum may contain other compounds. Ingredients may include other cannabinoids or terpenes, depending on the manufacturer and the quality of the oil.

Some CBD oil producers mix in a touch of these compounds

alongside CBD. They hypothesize that these compounds have an entourage effect, wherein their combined effects are more pronounced in the body.

Disorders characterized by convulsions and epileptic seizures

A seizure is an abnormal and brief increase in brain electrical activity. Seizures can be brought on by underlying conditions like epilepsy.

About 30% of people with epilepsy have difficulty controlling their symptoms using traditional methods. These patients should discuss the possibility of using CBD to treat their seizures with their physician.

To some extent, CBD may help reduce the frequency and severity of seizures. Nonetheless, learning more about cannabis is a slow process. Evidence suggests that CBD may help control seizures, but scientists have been hampered by government regulations surrounding cannabis, according to the Epilepsy Foundation.

Most countries and states still outlaw cannabis products with THC concentrations of 0.3% or higher. Epidolex, however, a drug containing CBD and classified as schedule V by the FDA, has been given the green light.

Although Epidolex is the only FDA-approved drug to utilize CBD, other products that contain CBD, such as oils and edibles, are legal across the United

States, provided they contain less than 0.3% THC.

Recently published studies lend credence to the idea that cannabidiol (CBD) products may be useful in treating some forms of epilepsy, thanks in large part to CBD's rescheduling.

However, researchers did not control the dosage or preparation of CBD in the majority of studies using CBD products, so researchers must continue to explore this area.

Please visit our CBD resource center for more details on this topic.

Both Lennox-Gastaut and Dravet syndromes

The rare forms of epilepsy known as Lennox-Gastaut syndrome and Dravet syndrome have drawn the attention of those who believe CBD may be especially helpful in these cases. Most cases of these syndromes manifest in young children; they are difficult to treat and can lead to life-threatening complications like seizures.

Some doctors prescribe the FDA-approved CBD isolate Epidiolex to treat the seizures that these rare forms of epilepsy cause.

In their report, they emphasize the significance of maintaining a constant dosage and administration schedule. This can give a person taking Epidiolex the confidence that they are getting the exact dose they need.

Epidiolex has about 98% pure CBD, making it more effective

and consistent than CBD isolates and oils.

According to anecdotal reports, people have used CBD and CBD oils to alleviate epilepsy and other symptoms.

Anyone thinking about trying out CBD or broad-spectrum oils should first consult with a medical professional.

cannabidiol (CBD) and children

CBD has shown promise in treating epilepsy in children, especially those whose symptoms have not responded to more traditional therapies. For those who are over the age of 2 and have been diagnosed with Lennox-Gastaut or Dravet syndrome, the FDA has approved the drug Epidiolex.

A review in the Journal of Clinical Neurophysiology notes that CBD, either isolated or part of a CBD-enriched herbal extract, helps decrease seizure frequency in children with treatment-resistant epilepsy.

Evidence suggests cannabidiol (CBD) reduces seizures in

children with drug-resistant epilepsy, according to a second review published in Epilepsia, but this effect does not generalize to other compounds in cannabis. CBD is widely believed to be the only compound with such desirable characteristics.

CBD may not be safe or effective for use in all children over the long term. Over the course of four years, CBD proved effective for about 27 percent of children with treatment-resistant epilepsy, according to a study published in CNS Drugs. While taking this medication, about 81% of participants reported some sort of adverse effect, with about 23% reporting serious problems.

Possible adverse effects

When considering CBD oil as a treatment for epilepsy or seizures, patients should be aware of a number of potential risks and side effects.

There are few, mild side effects associated with CBD oil use. There are a number of potential CBD-related side effects.

Feelings of drowsiness or exhaustion

• drowsiness

• diarrhea

• abdominal distress

Examples: • shifts in body mass

Preference shifts

It's possible that CBD could impair a person's ability to drive or operate heavy machinery.

Having thoughts of suicide

CBD use may be associated with an increased risk of suicidal thoughts in some people. One article in the year 2020 acknowledges a connection between the two, but stresses that CBD may not be to blame for this result.

CBD may be linked to an increase in suicidal thoughts, but more study is needed to confirm this. Users of CBD should keep an eye out for any strange symptoms or changes in behavior.

Prevention of Suicide

Someone you know may be in imminent danger of harming themselves or others if you do not intervene immediately.

Don't be afraid to ask, "Are you thinking about suicide?"

Don't pass judgment and just listen.

• To speak with a trained crisis counselor, call 911 or your local emergency number, or text TALK to 741741.

It's important that you stay with the person until help arrives.

It is recommended that you get rid of any weapons, medications, or other harmful items.

Potential harm to the liver

Some people taking CBD, especially in combination with other drugs, may experience an increased risk of liver damage. If you have liver damage and decide to use CBD, it's important to work with your doctor to keep an eye on your liver.

Substance-drug Interactions

CBD is a naturally occurring compound, but it could potentially interact with pharmaceuticals. Always consult your doctor before using CBD to rule out any potential side effects.

Grapefruit juice may counteract the effects of certain medications, such as those processed through the cytochrome P450 (CYP450) enzymatic pathway.

There are also possible dangers associated with using CBD.

It is also important for people to understand the relationship between various medications and supplements. Changes in blood levels are especially important to track for those with liver or renal disease.

The study of plant extracts and their potential interactions with pharmaceuticals is in its infancy.

However, some studies suggest that the following herbs may interact with CBD and other electrolytes via the CYP450 pathway:

Milk thistle

- echinacea

One example is the herb Ginkgo biloba.

- garlic

St. John's Wort

- goldenseal

Purity

When looking for CBD oil, it is essential to find a product with a high level of purity. This is of utmost importance to those who intend to use CBD oil as an adjunctive therapy for epilepsy and similar disorders.

Most reputable producers will provide lab results detailing the concentrations of compounds like CBD present in each bottle. This guarantees the most precise dosing possible.

A product's lack of chemical, pesticide, or heavy metal contamination can also be verified by means of an independent laboratory test.

You can rest assured that the quality of any CBD product featured on Medical News Today has been verified by an independent lab.

A test for drugs

Even though cannabidiol (CBD) is the main component of CBD

oil, small amounts of THC may be present. Although this quantity would not be sufficient to trigger a psychoactive effect in the brain, it may still register positive on a drug test.

Individuals using CBD for medical purposes who are subject to random drug testing should be aware of this possibility and take all necessary precautions.

CHAPTER THREE

Instructions for use

CBD oils are difficult to dose precisely, making oil purity all the more important.

Children and adults with Lennox-Gastaut syndrome who took 10 or 20 milligrams of CBD per kilogram of bodyweight per day in addition to their anti-epileptic medication experienced greater reductions in drop seizures, according to a study published in the New England Journal of Medicine.

The easiest way to administer CBD oil is probably by placing a drop or two under the tongue. If the person really doesn't like the taste, mixing it with some juice might do the trick.

However, anyone considering CBD to treat seizures and epilepsy should talk to their doctor about dosing, as it is important to find the minimum effective dose.

CHAPTER FOUR

Summary

CBD's therapeutic potential for treating seizures has grown as a result of recent scientific investigation. While cannabidiol (CBD) use has shown promise in helping some patients with treatment-resistant epilepsy, it isn't the best option for everyone.

Consult a medical professional in each instance to rule out any dangerous drug interactions and explore alternate treatment options. Those who opt for CBD should still keep in close contact with their physician to track progress and report any adverse reactions.

To back up the preliminary evidence that CBD may aid in the treatment of seizures, new high-quality studies can be conducted as legislation concerning CBD becomes more permissive.

www.ingramcontent.com/pod-product-compliance
Lightning Source LLC
La Vergne TN
LVHW010512160826
845677LV00012B/2802

9798847088343